ALOE VERA

MARIAN KIM

CONTENTS

MARIAN KIM

1

PROPERTIES

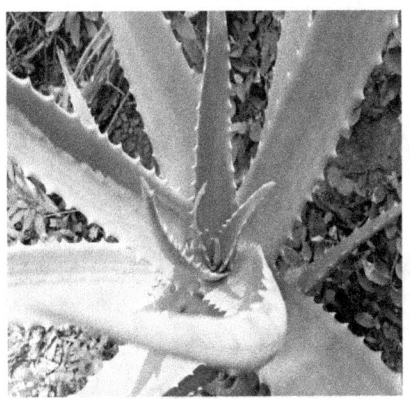

Scientific name: Aloe barbadensis, Aloe vera

Other names: Lily of the desert, burn plant

Nutrients: Vitamins A, B1, B2, B3, B6, B9 (folic acid), B12, C and E. Minerals like calcium, chromium, copper, magnesium, manganese, potassium, sodium, zinc and selenium. 7 of the 8 essential acids, water

Aloe vera gel also contains salicylic acid and 5 other antiseptics (e.g. sulfur and cinnamonic acid) which give it anti-bacterial, anti-viral and anti-fungal properties. Salicylic acid also has anti-inflammatory properties. Lignin is another very important component of aloe vera gel since it helps other products applied with the gel to the skin penetrate the skin better. It also contains phenolic compounds which absorb UV light and reduce the tendency to hyper-pigmentation (skin darkening).

Aloe Vera Properties

Anti-inflammatory properties

Antioxidant properties

Skin cell regenerating properties

Moisturizing

Antiseptic (antibacterial, antifungal, antiviral) properties

Skin soothing properties

Promotes wound healing

Immune stimulating properties

Stimulates collagen production

Stimulates hair growth

Absorbs UV light

* * * * *

2

USES

Aloe Vera Medically Proven Uses

Psoriasis treatment

Applying a 0.5% aloe vera cream for a month appears to lessen the plaque lesions of psoriasis.

Constipation treatment

Aloe vera contains compounds with a laxative effect and can therefore manage constipation by causing diarrhea. But since continued use of aloe laxatives can paralyze the walls on the intestines, these laxatives are no longer in the market.

Diabetes treatment

Aloe vera has been shown to lower blood glucose levels in patients with type 2 diabetics without any of the side effects associated with prescription medications used to treat diabetes.

***

Other Uses of Aloe Vera

Dry skin moisturization

Aloe vera gel is a wonderful moisturizer for dry skin since it contains over 90% water and has a great water holding capacity.

Sensitive skin soother

Aloe vera gel acts as a balm which soothes sensitive skin.

Acne treatment

Aloe vera contains salicylic acid which is used treat acne. It also has anti-inflammatory properties which are useful for managing the inflammation associated with acne. Its antiseptic properties are also useful for dealing with the acne causing bacteria. Aloe vera gel also acts as a soothing balm for inflamed skin. It also stimulates cell regeneration and is vital for the healing process. Since it is over 90% water, it is also an excellent oil free moisturizer. It also softens the skin and tightens the pores.

Eczema treatment

Aloe vera's gel anti-inflammatory and antipruritic properties are useful for managing the inflammation and itching of eczema. It is also an effective moisturizer which reduces the dryness associated with this condition.

Mature skin

Aloe vera increases the production of collagen and elastin fibers. This makes the skin more elastic and less wrinkled.

Prematurely aging skin

The potent antioxidants in aloe vera gel are useful for preventing and managing prematurely aging skin.

Itchy skin relief

The antipruritic properties of aloe vera gel reduce the itch.

Cold sore treatment

Aloe's antiviral properties are useful for managing cold sores or herpes skin infections.

Sunburns

Aloes skin regeneration properties help burns heal faster

First and second degree thermal burns

First degree thermal burns like kitchen burns were shown to heal faster after the application of aloe vera.

Radiation burns

Burns which developed after cancer patients received radiotherapy were also shown to heal faster after the application of aloe vera.

Electrical burns

Aloe vera's analgesic properties also help reduce the pain of burns.

Frostbite

General wounds and surgical wounds

Aloe vera has also been shown to promote wound healing through the production of collagen and elastin. It does this by stimulating fibroblasts which are the cells that produce them. Aloe vera can also improve the circulation of blood around a wound and thus accelerate its healing. Aloe vera also has antiseptic (antibacterial, antifungal, antiviral) properties which can also contribute to the faster healing of wounds by preventing infections.

Bedsores

Aloe vera helps all types of sores and wounds heal faster. It stimulates collagen production whichis vital for wound healing, increases the blood circulation and prevents infections. Its analgesic properties are also important since they reduce the pain.

Bruises

Aloe vera gel reduces the swelling associated with bruises.

Reduce scarring

Aloe vera contains compounds which help the skin heal faster and with minimal scarring

Managing inflamed skin

Aloe vera gel is used to manage inflamed skin because of its anti-inflammatory and skin soothing properties.

Hives treatment

Aloe gel is used to manage hives or urticaria and other allergic skin reactions.

Wart treatment

Aloe vera gel's antiviral properties are useful for helping warts heal.

Moisturizing dry scalps

Aloe vera gel is effective for moisturizing dry scalps and hair.

Managing inflamed scalp

Aloe vera gel is used to make products to manage inflamed scalps because of its anti-inflammatory properties and skin soothing properties.

Dandruff treatment

Alopecia or hair loss and thinning hair treatment since it stimulates hair growth

Lowering high cholesterol levels

Taking 10 ml or 20 ml of aloe vera by mouth for 3 months was shown to lower cholesterol levels in study participants with hyperlipidemia (high cholesterol levels). It also lowers triglyceride levels.

Managing ulcerative colitis

Taking 25 ml to 50 ml of aloe vera gel by mouth may reduce symptoms in persons with ulcerative colitis.

Crohn's disease treatment

Aloe vera gel is also used to manage Crohn's disease.

Irritable bowel syndrome (IBS) treatment

Aloe vera gel is used to reduce the symptoms of IBS.

Arthritis treatment

Aloe's anti-inflammatory properties are useful for managing joint inflammation and especially that of osteoarthritis.

Heart disease prevention

Aloe does this by making the blood less sticky

Stroke prevention

Aloe does this by making the blood less sticky

High blood pressure or hypertension treatment

Athlete's foot treatment

Aloe's antifungal properties are useful for managing fungal infections like athlete's foot.

Fungal infection prevention

Aloe has antifungal properties which are useful for preventing fungal infections like candida.

Intestinal worms removal

Aloe acts like a vermifuge and helps remove worms in the intestines.

Managing periodontitis

A study in the Journal of Ethnopharmacology revealed that aloe vera reduced the bleeding and swelling associated with these dental diseases. These effects can be attributed to its anti-inflammatory and antiseptic properties.

Preventing angular cheilitis

Aloe prevents wounds on the side of the mouth due to its to its antibacterial, antiviral and antifungal properties.

Preventing aphthous ulcers

Aloe prevents wounds inside the mouth due to its antibacterial, antiviral and antifungal properties.

Maintaining healthy teeth and gums

Managing gingivitis

Preventing denture stomatitis

Fever reducer

Aloe has antipyretic properties and it is thus able to reduce or prevent fevers.

Preventing degenerative diseases

By virtue of containing the potent anti-oxidants vitamins A, C, E and selenium, aloe vera is able to prevent degenerative diseases which have been attributed to free radical damage. These diseases include atherosclerosis, asthma, cancer, degenerative eye disease, diabetes, inflammatory joint disease and senile dementia.

Detoxifier

The gelatinous nature of aloe gel helps it mops up toxins in the gut and aid their excretion from the body.

General health booster

Aloe vera gel contains over 70 different vital nutrients. These include vitamins like vitamins A, B1, B2, B3 (niacin), B6, B9 (folic acid), B12, C and E. It also contains minerals like calcium, chromium, copper, iron, magnesium, manganese, potassium, selenium, sodium and zinc. 7 of the 8 essential amino acids are also found in this gel.

Heartburn and acid reflux treatment

Peptic ulcers treatment

Asthma treatment

Kidney stones prevention

Colon cancer prevention

Hemorrhoid treatment

The uses of aloe vera also extend to the natural management of hemorrhoids. Its astringent and pain relieving properties are useful when it is applied directly to the hemorrhoids. Its constipation relieving properties are also important when it is taken by mouth since constipation is one of the causative factors for hemorrhoids.

Stretch marks reducer

Aloe vera gel is said to reduce the appearance of stretch marks.

Razor burn reducer

When used as a shaving gel, aloe vera gel can reduce razor burns and help minor cuts heal faster and with less scarring.

Oily skin moisturizer

Aloe vera gel does not contain oil and it is thus perfect for moisturizing oily and acne prone skin.

Alopecia or hair loss treatment

Aloe is used for alopecia since it stimulates hair growth.

Frizzy hair management

Aloe vera gel can be used as a hair gel to reduce frizz and keep flyaway hairs in their place.

Seborrheic dermatitis treatment

Insect bites

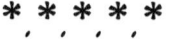

3

SAFETY PRECAUTIONS

1. Do not drink aloe vera gel or juice if you are pregnant or breastfeeding or menstruating.

2. Do not take aloe vera gel by mouth if you are scheduled to have surgery within two weeks since it can cause prolonged bleeding.

3. Aloe vera may cause redness, stinging and burning sensations on the application site. A few cases of contact dermatitis have also been reported.

4. If you are allergic to allium family foods like onions and garlic, it is best not to use aloe vera gel since you may develop itching, hives and even more severe allergic reactions.

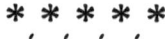

4

DRUG INTERACTIONS

1. Do not use/avoid aloe vera if you are taking glyburide which is used to treat diabetes since they both can lower blood glucose levels.

2. Do not use/avoid aloe vera if you are taking diuretics (water pills) since they can both reduce levels of potassium in the body.

3. Do not use/avoid aloe vera if you are taking digoxin since they can both reduce levels of potassium in the body.

4. Do not apply aloe vera gel to the skin if you are applying hydrocortisone since it can increase the effectiveness of this corticosteroid cream.

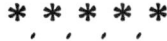

5

TIPS

Buy an organic aloe vera plant and cut off one leaf. Scoop the gel from the leaf and use it for your herbal recipes. Store the cut leaf in the refrigerator until you have used all its gel.

6

HERBAL RECIPES

Aloe Vera Juice

Equipment

Glass jar with tight fitting lid

Sharp knife

Spoon

Plate

Blender

***

Ingredients

Organic aloe vera plant

***

Instructions

1. Cut a leaf or two from an organic aloe vera plant. Pick the mature leaves at the bottom.

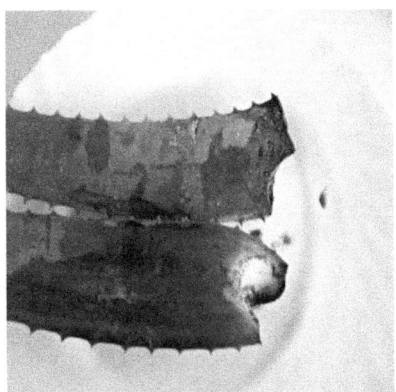

2. Make the leaves stand in the jar for at least 15 minutes to drain the resin completely

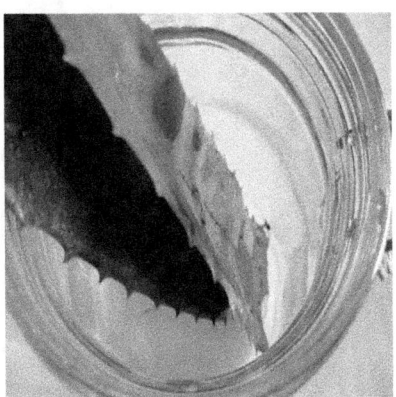

3. Wash the leaves

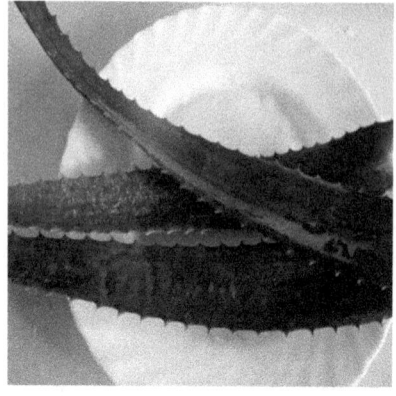

4. Cut off the thorns from both sides of the leaves

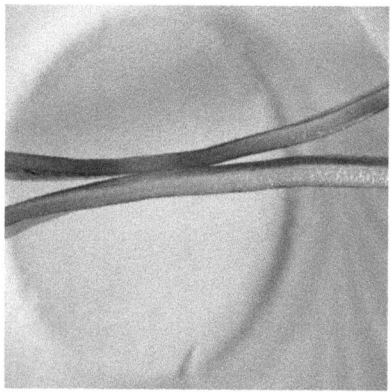

5. Cut the leaves lengthwise in the middle.

6. Scoop out the gel with a clean spoon ensuring that it does not have any yellow or green parts.

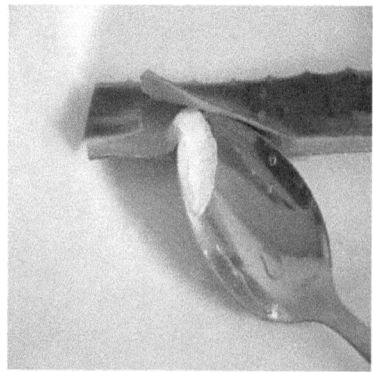
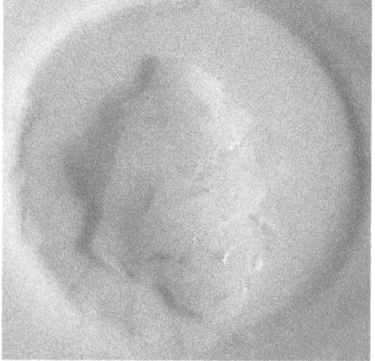

7. Blend 2 tablespoons of the aloe vera gel with a glass of water for around 3 minutes to make organic aloe vera juice.

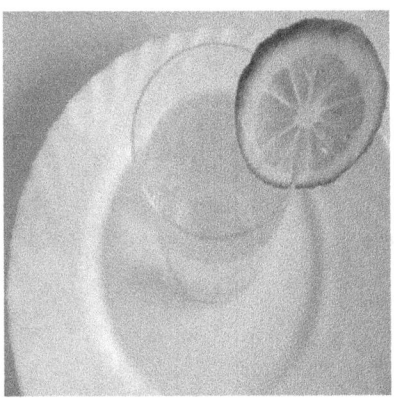

***

Tips

1. Drink the aloe vera juice immediately after making it since its medicinal benefits are reduced once it gets oxidized and this can happen while it is stored in the refrigerator.

2. You can sweeten the aloe vera juice with honey if you find it bitter.

3. You can also blend the aloe vera gel with fruit juices like orange and lemon. You can also blend it with coconut milk and almond milk.

*****

Aloe Vera Fruit Smoothie

Equipment
Blender

***

Recipe Ingredients
1 cup aloe vera juice

2 cups banana slices

1 cup mango slices

6 medium ice cubes

Honey to taste (optional)

***

Instructions
Put all the ingredients in a blender and puree for a few minutes until you get a smooth consistency.

Serve immediately.

***

Tip
You can increase or decrease the amount of aloe vera juice to decrease or increase the consistency of the smoothie.

*****

Aloe Vera Green Smoothie

Equipment

Blender

***

Recipe Ingredients

4 cups aloe vera juice

2 cups baby spinach leaves

1 cup banana slices

Honey to taste (optional)

***

Instructions

Put all the ingredients in a blender and puree for a few minutes until you get a smooth consistency.

Serve immediately.

***

Tip

You can increase or decrease the amount of aloe vera juice to decrease or increase the consistency of the smoothie.

*****

Aloe Vera Milk

Equipment

Blender

***

Recipe Ingredients

4 cups aloe vera juice

1 cup banana slices

I cup almonds

***

Instructions

Put all the ingredients in a blender and puree for a few minutes until you get a smooth consistency.

Serve immediately.

***

Tip

You can increase or decrease the amount of aloe vera juice to decrease or increase the consistency of the smoothie.

*****

Aloe Vera Lotion

Equipment
Double boiler

***

Ingredients
1 cup aloe vera gel

1/2 cup beeswax, grated

1/3 cup vegetable oil like olive oil or sweet almond oil

10 drops essential oils like lavender (optional natural fragrance)

1 teaspoon vitamin E oil (optional natural preservative)

***

Instructions
1. Mix the beeswax and the vegetable oil in a glass bowl and place it in a double boiler to melt the beeswax. You can also melt it in the microwave by heating it for 30 second bursts.

2. Mix the aloe vera, vitamin E and essential oil in another bowl.

3. Pour the melted beeswax mixture into the blender and turn it to low. Pour in the aloe vera mixture slowly.

4. Once it is well mixed pour the lotion into clean jars.

*****

Aloe Vera Acne Treatment Gel

Equipment

Dark jar with large mouth and tight fitting lid

***

Recipe Ingredients

95 ml aloe vera gel

5 ml tea tree essential oil

***

Instructions

1. Mix all the ingredients together in the jar with the large mouth.

***

Tips

A study conducted at the Royal Prince Alfred proved that a 5% tea tree gel is effective for the treatment of mild to moderate acne.

*****

Aloe Vera Moisturizer

Equipment

Dark jar with tight fitting lid

***

Ingredients

1 cup aloe vera gel

1 tablespoon vegetable oil like olive oil or sweet almond oil

1 teaspoon vitamin E

10 drops essential oils like lavender or geranium

***

Instructions

1. Mix all the ingredients in the dark jar with a tight fitting lid.

***

Tips

1. Store the aloe vera moisturizer in the refrigerator to prolong its shelf life.

2. To make a moisturizer for eczema use evening primrose oil as your vegetable oil and Roman chamomile as your essential oil.

###

ABOUT THE AUTHOR

Marian Kim is an experienced alternative medicine practitioner.

*****

OTHER BOOKS BY THE AUTHOR

ALLSPICE

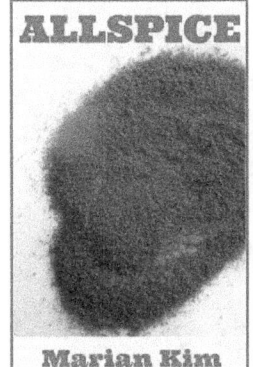

Marian Kim

ALOE VERA

Marian Kim

BASIL

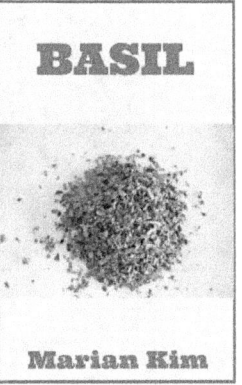

Marian Kim

BAY LEAF

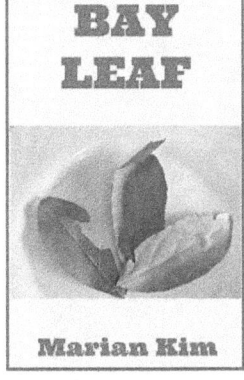

Marian Kim

CALENDULA

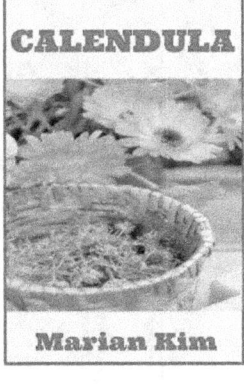

Marian Kim

CARDAMOM

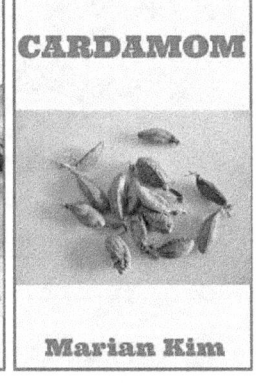

Marian Kim

CAYENNE PEPPER

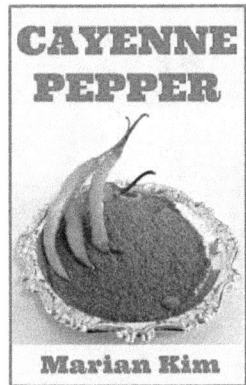

Marian Kim

CHAMOMILE

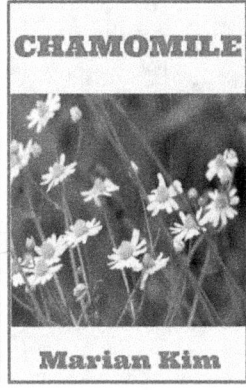

Marian Kim

CILANTRO & CORIANDER

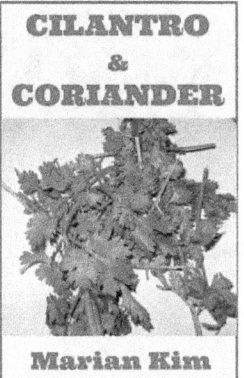

Marian Kim

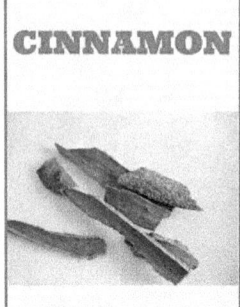
CINNAMON
Marian Kim

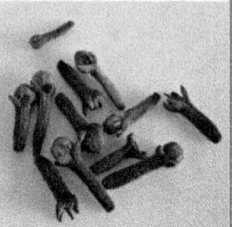
CLOVES
Marian Kim

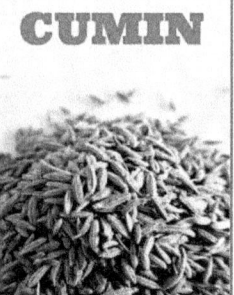
CUMIN
Marian Kim

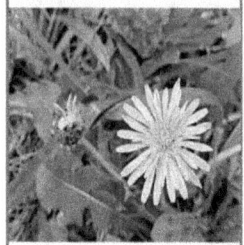
DANDELION
Marian Kim

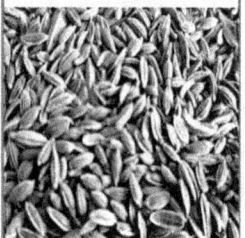
DILL
Marian Kim

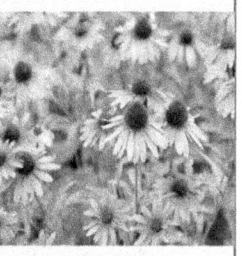
ECHINACEA
Marian Kim

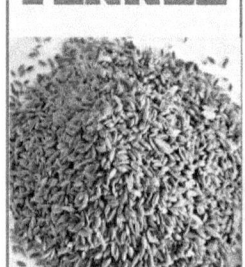
FENNEL
Marian Kim

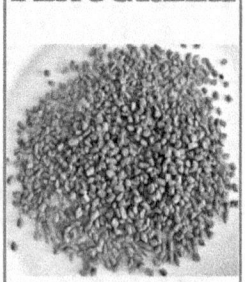
FENUGREEK
Marian Kim

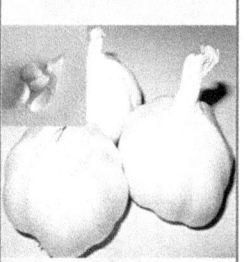
GARLIC
Marian Kim

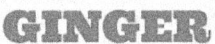

GINGER

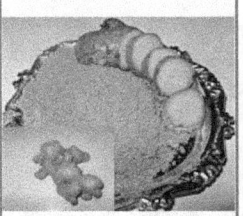

Marian Kim

GINKGO BILOBA

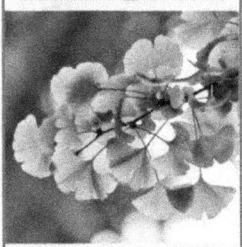

Marian Kim

GINSENG

Marian Kim

LAVENDER

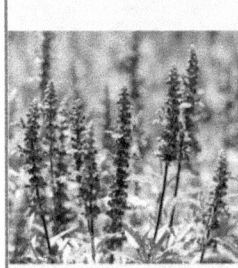

Marian Kim

MUSTARD

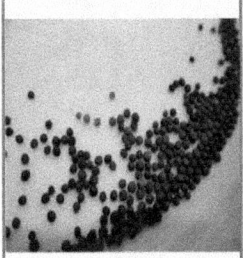

Marian Kim

NEEM

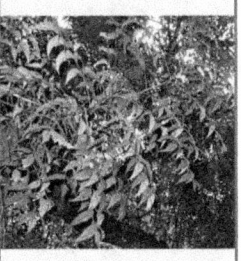

Marian Kim

NUTMEG & MACE

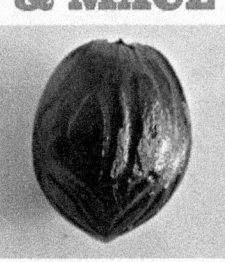

Marian Kim

OREGANO

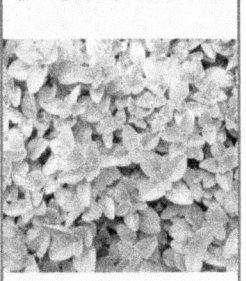

Marian Kim

PAPRIKA

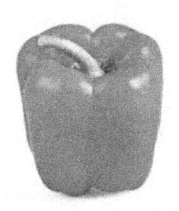

Marian Kim

PARSLEY

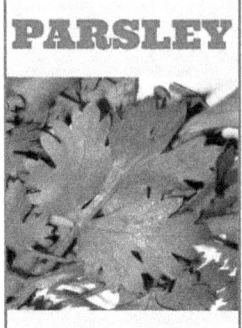

Marian Kim

BLACK & WHITE PEPPER

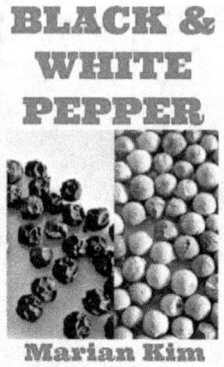

Marian Kim

PEPPERMINT

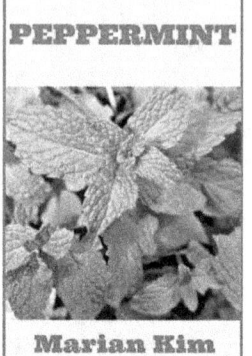

Marian Kim

ROSE HIPS

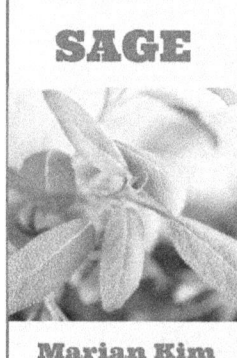

Marian Kim

ROSE PETALS

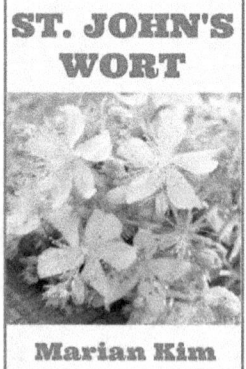

Marian Kim

ROSEMARY

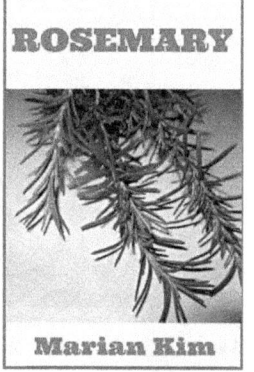

Marian Kim

SAGE

Marian Kim

ST. JOHN'S WORT

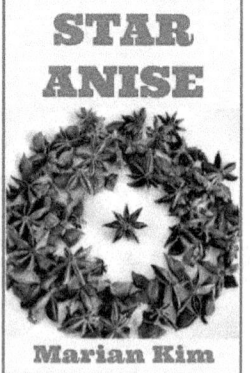

Marian Kim

STAR ANISE

Marian Kim

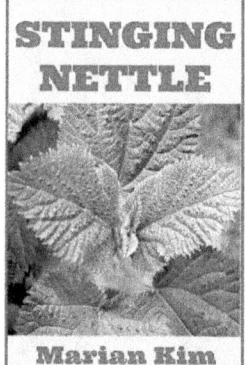

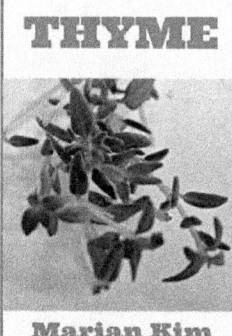

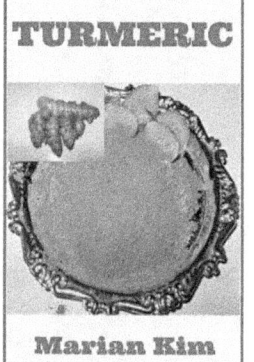

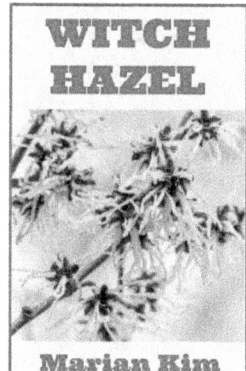

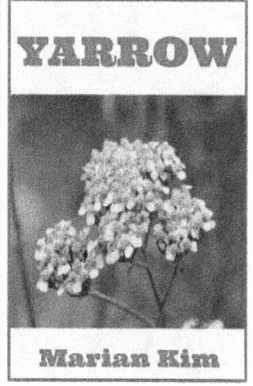

*****